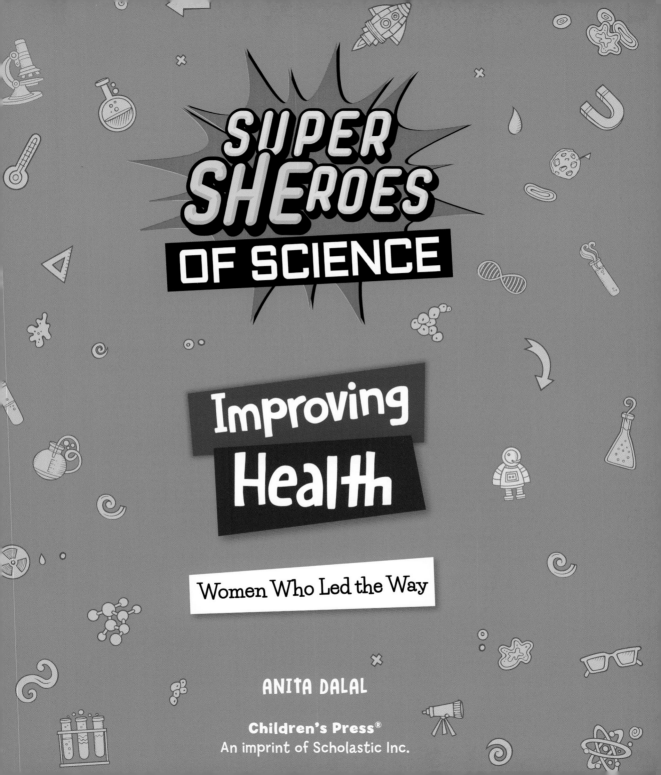

Super SHEROES

OF SCIENCE

Improving Health

Women Who Led the Way

ANITA DALAL

Children's Press®
An imprint of Scholastic Inc.

Library of Congress Cataloging-in-Publication Data

Names: Dalal, Anita, author.

Title: Improving health : women led the way / Anita Dalal.

Description: First edition. | New York, NY : Children's Press, an imprint of Scholastic Inc.,
2022. | Series: Super SHEroes of science | Includes bibliographical references and
index. | Audience: Ages 8–10 | Audience: Grades 4–6 | Summary: "Audience: Ages 8–10. | Audience: Grades 4–6. |
Summary: "This brand-new series highlights some of the major contributions women have made in the world of
science. Photographs throughout"— Provided by publisher.

Identifiers: LCCN 2021037456 (print) | LCCN 2021037457 (ebook) | ISBN
9781338800340 (library binding) | ISBN 9781338800357 (paperback) | ISBN
9781338800371 (ebk)

Subjects: LCSH: Women in medicine--Biography--Juvenile literature. | Women
in science--Biography--Juvenile literature. | Women in
medicine--History--Juvenile literature. | Women in
science--History--Juvenile literature. | BISAC: JUVENILE NONFICTION /
Biography & Autobiography / Women

Classification: LCC R692 .D35 2022 (print) | LCC R692 (ebook) | DDC
610.922 [B]--dc23

LC record available at https://lccn.loc.gov/2021037456

LC ebook record available at https://lccn.loc.gov/2021037457

Picture credits:

Photos ©: cover top: Jemal Countess/Getty Images; cover center top: Courtesy of the Helen Rodríguez-Trías Papers/ Archives of the Puerto Rican Diaspora/Center for Puerto Rican Studies/Hunter College City University of New York; cover center bottom: Yang Wumin Xinhua/eyevine/Redux; cover bottom: Pictorial Press Ltd/Alamy Images; 5 left: Jemal Countess/Getty Images; 5 center left: Courtesy of the Helen Rodríguez-Trías Papers/ Archives of the Puerto Rican Diaspora/Center for Puerto Rican Studies/Hunter College City University of New York; 5 center right: Pictorial Press Ltd/Alamy Images; 5 right: Yang Wumin Xinhua/eyevine/Redux; 6 inset top: Colport/Alamy Images; 6 right: North Wind Picture Archives/Alamy Images; 7 top: Jonathan Brady/Getty Images; 7 bottom: lucky-photographer/ Getty Images; 8 top: Look and Learn/Bridgeman Images; 9 top: Amoret Tanner/Alamy Images; 10 bottom: Science History Images/Alamy Images; 11 top: British Library Board. All Rights Reserved/Bridgeman Images; 12 inset top: agefotostock/Alamy Images; 13 top right: Interim Archives/Getty Images; 15 top: John Parrot/Stocktrek Images/Getty Images; 16 bottom: Corbis Historical/Getty Images; 17 top: Hulton-Deutsch Collection/Corbis/Getty Images; 18 top left: Schlesinger Library, Radcliffe Institute, Harvard/Bridgeman Images; 20 inset top: Pictorial Press Ltd/Alamy Images; 21 top: National Archives and Records Administration; 22 top: Glasshouse Images/Shutterstock; 26 top: University of Hawaii at Manoa/Colorization by Jacqueline Moore Chun; 27 bottom left: Sepia Times/Universal Images Group/ Getty Images; 28 inset top: Yang Wumin Xinhua/eyevine/Redux; 30 top: ADN-Bildarchiv/ullstein bild/Getty Images; 31 top: James Wheeler/500px/Getty Images; 32 bottom right: 4X-image/Getty Images; 33 center: Soren Andersson/AFP/Getty Images; 34 top: North Wind Picture Archives/Alamy Images; 35 top: Harold Clements/Daily Express/Hulton Archive/Getty Images; 36 top: Sarin Images/The Granger Collection; 36 bottom: Bettmann/Getty Images; 37 top: Courtesy of the Helen Rodríguez-Trías Papers/ Archives of the Puerto Rican Diaspora/Center for Puerto Rican Studies/Hunter College City University of New York; 37 bottom: Kimberly White/Reuters/Alamy Images; 38 top: Jemal Countess/Getty Images; 39 top: Steve Parsons/Press Association/AP Images; 40 top left: Everett Collection Inc/ Alamy Images; 40 top right: Shawshots/Alamy Images; 40 bottom left: Fine Art Images/Heritage Images/Getty Images; 41 bottom left: Science History Images/Alamy Images; 41 bottom center: Monika Graff/UPI/Newscom; 42–43: pop_jop/Getty Images; 44 top: Colport/ Alamy Images; 44 center: agefotostock/Alamy Images; 44 bottom right: Yang Wumin Xinhua/eyevine/Redux; 45 bottom: Courtesy of the Helen Rodríguez-Trías Papers/ Archives of the Puerto Rican Diaspora/Center for Puerto Rican Studies/Hunter College City University of New York.

All other photos © Shutterstock.

10 9 8 7 6 5 4 3 2 1   22 23 24 25 26

Printed in the U.S.A. 113
First edition, 2022
Series produced for Scholastic by Parcel Yard Press

Contents

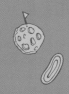

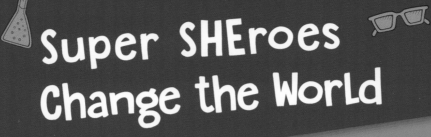

Super SHEroes Change the World

Women scientists, engineers, and inventors have made remarkable breakthroughs for centuries. Often, however, their achievements went unrecognized. Today far more women work in these fields than ever before, and their achievements are celebrated.

This book celebrates the life and the work of twelve of these women, twelve Super SHEroes of Science! They all worked, or still work, to improve health.

Health has to do with understanding and treating sickness in order to be free from disease. It also involves the well-being of communities.

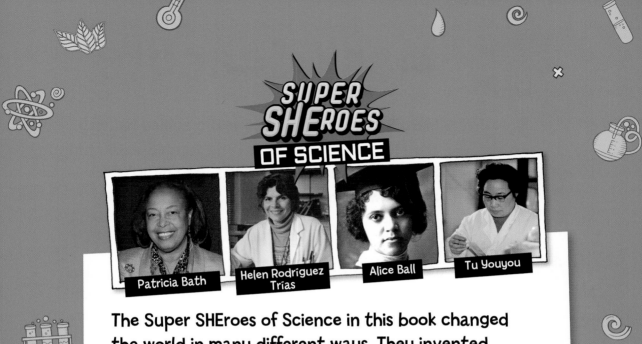

SUPER SHEROES OF SCIENCE

Patricia Bath

Helen Rodriguez Trias

Alice Ball

Tu Youyou

The Super SHEroes of Science in this book changed the world in many different ways. They invented treatments for eye problems, campaigned to improve health care, and found new cures for serious diseases. And many of these women started off by being told that science wasn't for them. But they stuck to their dreams, asked questions, and took risks. They eventually got to write their own stories.

This book brings their stories to you! And while you read them, remember:

Your story can change the world, too! You can become a Super SHEro of Science.

Mary Seacole

Mary Seacole was a nurse who traveled halfway around the world to care for wounded soldiers in Europe. At the time, that was very unusual for a Black woman.

SUPER SHERO OF SCIENCE

Mary was born on the Caribbean island of Jamaica to a Scottish father and a Jamaican mother. Mary's mom was a healer. She taught Mary traditional Jamaican medicine, which used many local herbs. Mary used to practice treating her dolls, dogs, cats, and even herself.

datafile

Born: 1805

Died: 1881

Place of birth: Jamaica

Field: Nursing

Super SHEro for: Saving the lives of people in the Caribbean and in the Crimea

Mary's mom ran a lodging house where she looked after sick and injured soldiers, and Mary often helped out.

In her teens, Mary traveled to London, England. She watched doctors there and learned about how they worked. She spent another two years in London a little later. Then she returned home to Kingston, the capital of Jamaica.

This memorial to Mary stands in London, England.

When Mary was born, Jamaica was governed by Great Britain.

At the age of thirty, Mary got married, but her husband, Edwin Seacole, was in poor health. Mary took care of him until he died eight years later. Mary was heartbroken, but when the deadly disease cholera broke out in Kingston, she offered to nurse victims.

What's Your Story?

?

Mary looked after patients suffering from serious diseases. The diseases spread easily in ways that people did not really understand at the time. Mary risked becoming very sick herself.

Have you ever put yourself at risk to help others?

Do you know other people who would put themselves at risk to help others?

Mary also looked after people during other epidemics. When yellow fever broke out in Kingston, Mary turned her mom's lodging house into a hospital for sick British soldiers. She nursed the soldiers, bathed them, and gave them healthy food.

When Britain and other countries went to war against Russia in 1853, Mary wanted to help. The war was mainly fought on the Crimean Peninsula on the Black Sea, which lies between Russia and Turkey.

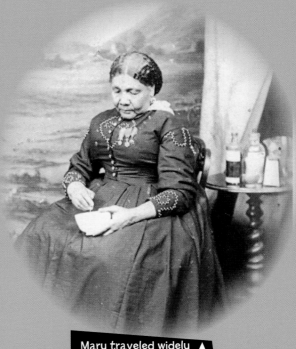

Mary traveled widely to help others.

Did You Know?

Diseases spread in different ways. Some, such as cholera, are spread by dirty water. Others, including malaria, are spread by insect bites. Diseases such as flu are spread by tiny droplets in the air. Wearing masks protects people from airborne diseases.

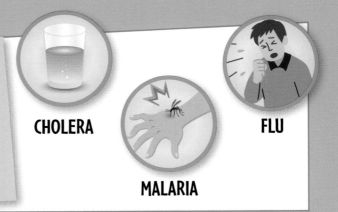

CHOLERA

MALARIA

FLU

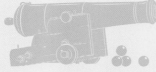

Mary traveled to London. She asked the War Office if she could go to Crimea to help British soldiers. The War Office refused, but she decided to go anyway. When she got to Crimea, she used her own money to set up the British Hotel. Wounded and sick soldiers used it to recover.

The hotel was much closer to the fighting than a hospital that had been set up for soldiers by the British nurse Florence Nightingale in Turkey. That meant Mary could go onto the battlefield, even under fire, to nurse wounded men. The soldiers called her "Mother Seacole."

Soldiers relaxed at the British Hotel as they recovered from their wounds.

When Mary returned to London after the war, she had no money left. The soldiers she had helped held a fundraiser for her, and 80,000 people turned up! Mary also wrote her autobiography to raise money. The *Wonderful Adventures of Mrs. Seacole* was a bestseller.

Mary died in 1881 and was soon forgotten about in Britain—but not in Jamaica. More than a hundred years later nurses visiting Britain from the Caribbean reminded people about Mary's remarkable career. **Thanks to them, Mary is now seen as a pioneer for nursing the sick and wounded.**

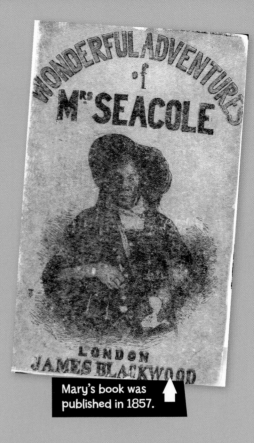

Mary's book was published in 1857.

What Would You Do?

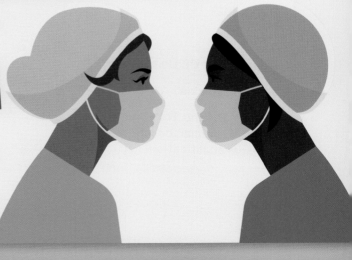

Mary was very brave. She did not give up when she was told she could not go to Crimea.

How would you make sure you could do something that really matters to you?

Mary was as famous as Florence Nightingale while she was alive, but she was soon forgotten.

What would you do if you discovered a forgotten Super SHEro of science?

Elizabeth Blackwell

In 1849, Elizabeth Blackwell was the first woman in the United States to become a doctor.

Elizabeth was born into a wealthy family in England. When she was eleven years old, her family moved to the United States. Unusually for the time, her parents hired private tutors to educate Elizabeth and her sisters. After Elizabeth's father died when she was just seventeen, she and her sisters opened a school to earn money. Elizabeth later worked as a teacher for a few years.

datafile

Born: 1821

Died: 1910

Place of birth: United Kingdom

Field: Medicine

Super SHEro for: Being the first woman doctor with a medical qualification

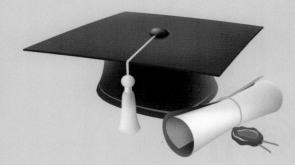

While Elizabeth was teaching, one of her friends was dying. The friend told Elizabeth she would have preferred her doctor to be a woman. Her words inspired Elizabeth to study medicine.

Elizabeth was rejected by many medical schools before she finally got a place. Once she was enrolled, she faced a lot of hostility because she was a woman. Despite that, she graduated head of the class.

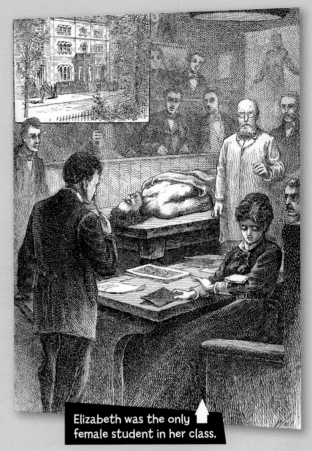

Elizabeth was the only female student in her class.

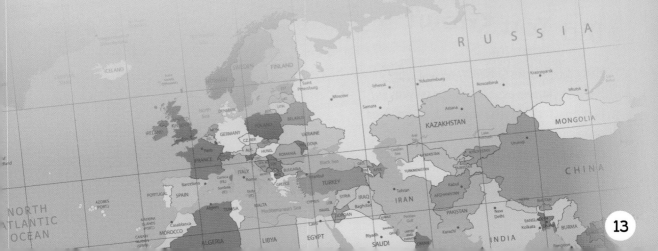

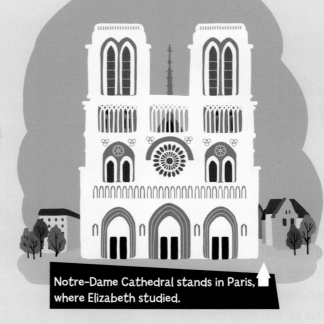

Notre-Dame Cathedral stands in Paris, where Elizabeth studied.

After she graduated from medical school, Elizabeth returned to Europe. She continued her studies in Paris. There, Elizabeth got an infection that left her blind in one eye. The infection ended her dream of becoming a surgeon. Surgeons need excellent eyesight.

Did You Know?

Many diseases are caused by certain types of microbes, known as germs. It was only in 1847 that a doctor in Austria noticed a link between cleanliness and disease. Washing his hands and cleaning wounds well reduced the spread of disease.

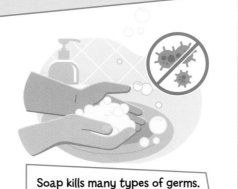

Soap kills many types of germs.

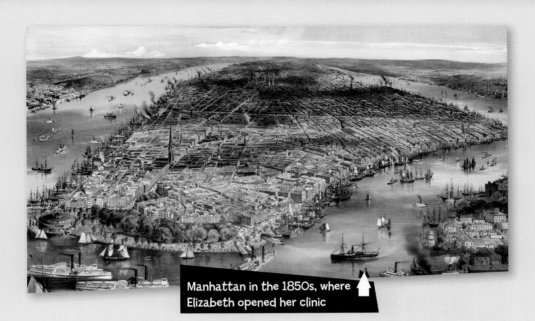

Manhattan in the 1850s, where Elizabeth opened her clinic

Back in New York in summer 1851, no hospital would hire Elizabeth because she was a woman. She even struggled to rent offices to practice as a private doctor.

In 1853, with the help of friends, she opened a small clinic in a very poor part of the city. Elizabeth worked there with her younger sister, Emily, who was also a doctor. They were joined by another female doctor, Marie Zakrzewska.

What's Your Story?

?

Elizabeth was a mentor to Marie Zakrzewska. Marie had come to the United States from Poland to train as a doctor. Elizabeth encouraged Marie and gave her a job in her clinic.

Has anyone been a mentor to you? How did they help you?

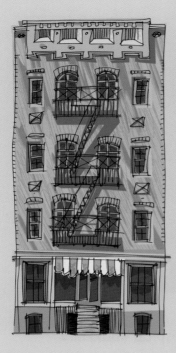

Elizabeth noticed that the women and children who came to the clinic were continually sick. Their homes were crowded and dirty. Elizabeth began to campaign for better living conditions. She thought this would improve people's health.

In 1857, along with Emily and Marie, Elizabeth opened a hospital for poor women and children in New York. As well as treating the poor, the hospital trained nurses.

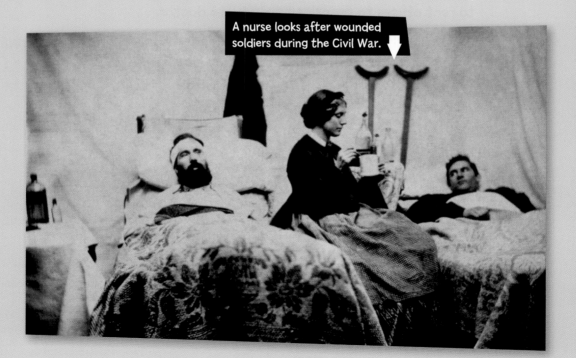

A nurse looks after wounded soldiers during the Civil War.

When the Civil War broke out in 1861, Elizabeth helped train nurses to look after wounded Union soldiers. After the war ended in 1865, she set up a women's medical college. Elizabeth only admitted the smartest students. She believed women doctors should be just as talented as male doctors.

Elizabeth's health got worse. She was forced to give up medicine in the 1870s and returned to England. She continued to campaign for better living conditions for the poor. **Today, Elizabeth's approach of trying to prevent disease by improving people's quality of life is used around the world.**

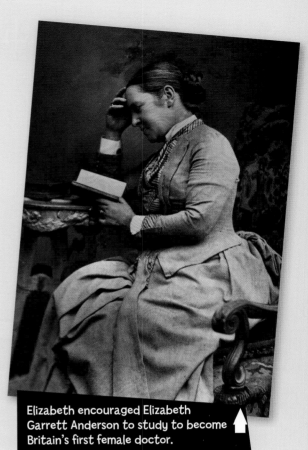

Elizabeth encouraged Elizabeth Garrett Anderson to study to become Britain's first female doctor.

What Would You Do?

Elizabeth became too sick to continue seeing patients. But she still helped people through improving living conditions.

What would you do if you could not do your first choice of career?

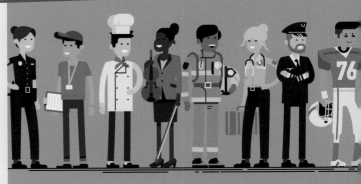

At Work with Elizabeth Blackwell

Elizabeth opened her clinic in a poor part of New York City that was home to a large immigrant community. Discover how she helped improve their health.

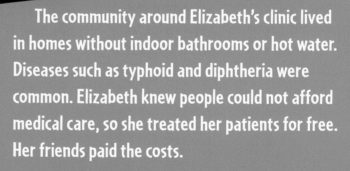

Elizabeth wanted to help the poor.

The community around Elizabeth's clinic lived in homes without indoor bathrooms or hot water. Diseases such as typhoid and diphtheria were common. Elizabeth knew people could not afford medical care, so she treated her patients for free. Her friends paid the costs.

Elizabeth's clinic opened at 3:00 p.m. every Monday, Wednesday, and Friday afternoon. It was a room in a house where the walls were lined with glass bottles containing a range of different tablets, powders, and liquids used as medicines.

Elizabeth at work

Elizabeth would examine the patient and ask them about their **symptoms**. She would then decide what she thought was wrong with them and give them the appropriate medicine.

To keep up with advances in medicine, Elizabeth read widely from medical books. When she lived in Paris, Elizabeth had a chance to use a new invention, the stethoscope. Invented in 1816, this long tube was used to listen to a patient's heart. Doctors could tell a lot about a person's health from their heartbeat.

Places of work: clinic, hospital, home study

Daily activities: seeing patients, reading, preparing medicines, fundraising

Main equipment: stethoscope, medicines

Main collaborators: Emily Blackwell and Marie Zakrzewska

Medicines

Stethoscope

Alice Ball

Alice Ball invented a new treatment for a serious disease called leprosy, but did not get credit for it.

Alice was born in Seattle, Washington, the third of four children. Her grandfather, J. P. Ball, was one of the first Americans to make early photographs, called daguerreotypes. Alice's father became a photographer, too, and so did her mother. When Alice was ten, her grandfather got sick. The family moved to Honolulu, Hawaii, in the hope that the sunny weather would help him.

datafile

Born: 1892

Died: 1916

Place of birth: United States

Field: Chemistry

Super SHEro for: Developing the first successful treatment for leprosy, the "Ball Method"

Alice's grandfather died two years later, and the family moved back to Seattle, where Alice went to high school. After she graduated in 1910 with top grades in science, she went to the University of Washington. There, she studied pharmacy, or how to prepare drugs for medical use.

Alice wrote a long article about medicine for the *Journal of the American Chemical Society*. At the time, such journals rarely had articles by women. For a Black woman to be published in the journal was a remarkable achievement.

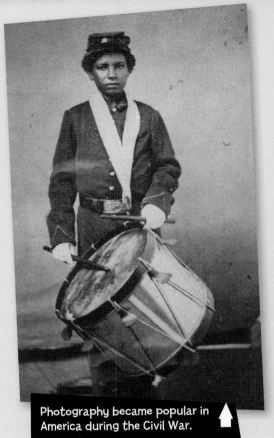

Photography became popular in America during the Civil War.

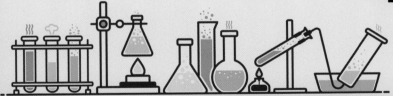

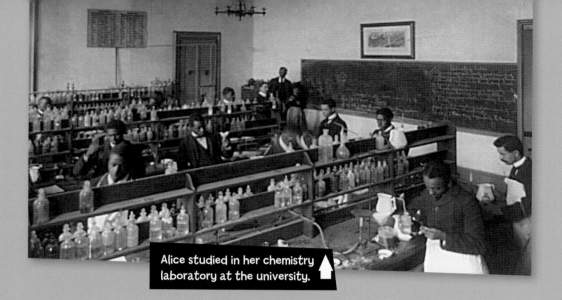

Alice studied in her chemistry laboratory at the university.

After Alice graduated, many universities offered her places to continue her graduate studies. She decided to return to Hawaii and study for a master's degree in chemistry. She graduated in 1915. She was the first ever Black woman at the University of Hawaii to be awarded a master's degree. Alice studied the chemistry of plants that grew on Pacific islands.

What's Your Story?

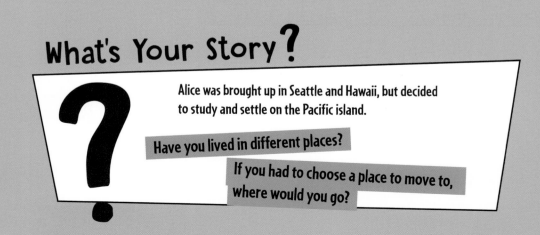

Alice was brought up in Seattle and Hawaii, but decided to study and settle on the Pacific island.

Have you lived in different places?

If you had to choose a place to move to, where would you go?

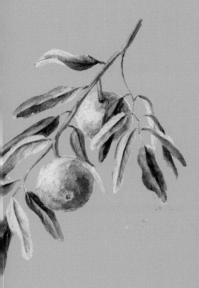

Alice met a Hawaiian doctor named Harry T. Hollmann. Hollmann was trying to isolate the chemicals in the chaulmoogra plant from India. Chaulmoogra oil was used in traditional medicine to treat leprosy, a disease that seriously affected the nerves and skin. When the oil was injected into patients, however, it caused side effects, including pain. People who swallowed it usually threw up.

Leprosy is caused by tiny germs.

Did You Know?

In many countries around the world, people rely on herbal remedies. The leaves, bark, flowers, and roots of plants are used as cures. Many modern drugs are based on plants.

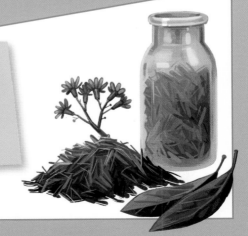

Harry Hollmann asked Alice to help him. Alice was teaching chemistry at the university, but in her spare time, she started to figure out a way to make the oil easier to use. Even though her time was limited, she solved the problem within a year. She used chaulmoogra oil to produce a **compound** that the body could absorb easily. Alice's method was revolutionary, but she died before she could publish her discovery. She was just twenty-four. Some people believe she may have been accidentally poisoned by chemicals at work.

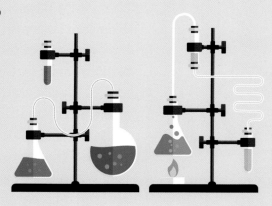

Today, about 210,000 people suffer from leprosy around the world, mainly in Africa and Asia.

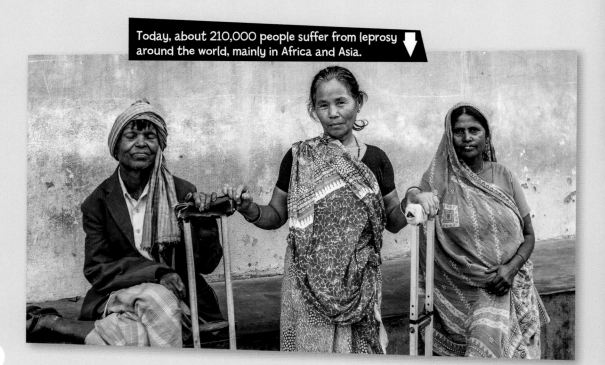

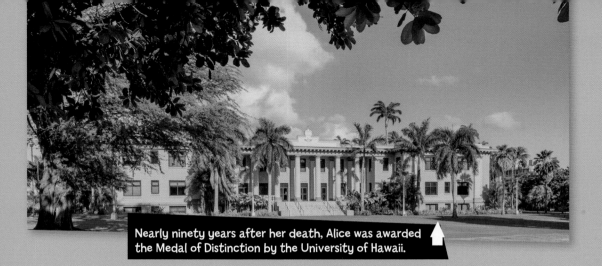

Nearly ninety years after her death, Alice was awarded the Medal of Distinction by the University of Hawaii.

Another chemist, Arthur L. Dean, published Alice's findings as his own. He went into business making the compound she had discovered. But Harry Hollmann knew Alice Ball had invented the cure. When he wrote an article in a medical journal about the cure, he called it the "Ball Method." That made sure Alice got credit for her invention. **Despite Hollmann's efforts, Alice was largely forgotten—but today she is finally getting the recognition she deserves.**

What Would You Do ?

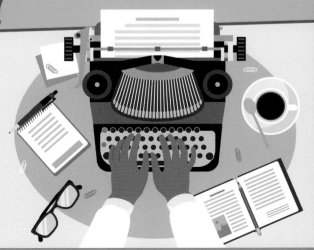

Harry Hollmann wanted the world to know that Alice, not Arthur Dean, had discovered the cure for leprosy. So, he wrote about it.

What would you do to right a wrong?

How would you go about it?

Alice wearing her academic robes

When Alice was alive, leprosy was a deadly disease with no known cure. Many patients lived on their own in communities, called colonies, until they died. Read about how Alice transformed their lives through her technique.

Although chaulmoogra oil helped treat the disease, it was difficult to apply. The oil was not soluble, meaning it did not dissolve in water, which made it hard for the body to absorb.

Alice did her research for Harry Hollmann in the evenings. She was determined to find a compound that the body could absorb easily. This problem had defeated other chemists, but Alice made a breakthrough.

Alice at work

She started by extracting the oil from the seeds of the chaulmoogra plant. Then she froze part of the oil overnight. This gave the chemicals she needed the right conditions to separate from the oil. Now she could turn them into a medicine!

Alice's work improved the lives of thousands of people with leprosy. The "Ball Method" was used successfully to treat patients for the next thirty years, until even more effective drugs were introduced.

Places of work: Lab at the University of Hawaii

Daily activities: teaching, carrying out experiments

Main equipment: test tubes, Bunsen burner, freezer

Major collaborators: Harry T. Hollmann

Test tubes

Bunsen burner

Lepers in Hawaii were sent to the island of Molokai.

MOLOKAI

Tu Youyou

Tu Youyou is a Chinese chemist who discovered a cure for malaria. This deadly disease kills between one and three million people every year.

SUPER SHEro OF SCIENCE

Tu Youyou was born in 1930 in the city of Ningbo on the east coast of China. When she was sixteen, she got the disease tuberculosis. She missed two years of school. When she recovered, she decided to study medicine. She wanted to help people by finding cures for diseases like the one she had suffered.

datafile

Born: 1930

Place of birth: China

Field: Chemistry

Super SHEro for: Discovering a treatment for malaria and winning the Nobel Prize

28

Tu went to medical college. She learned about medicinal plants and how to extract their ingredients and figure out their chemical structures. After she graduated, Tu joined the Academy of Traditional Chinese Medicine. She spent three years studying traditional Chinese cures. She spent the rest of her career as a researcher at the academy.

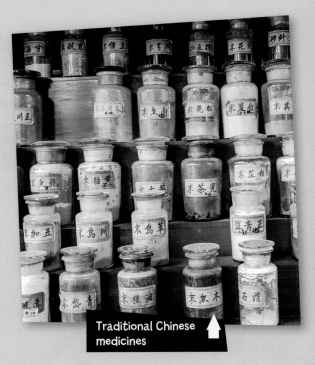

Traditional Chinese medicines

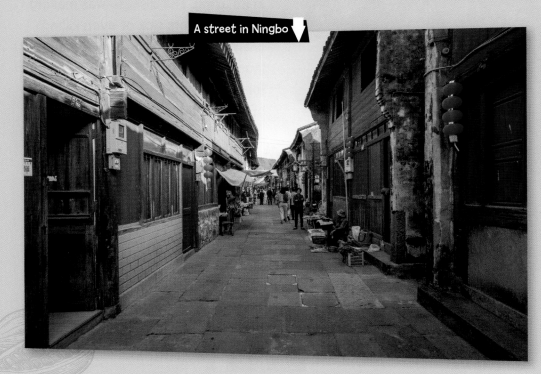

A street in Ningbo

What's Your Story?

?

While she was carrying out her research, Tu traveled a lot and missed spending time with her two children.

Have you ever had to miss something you really wanted to do because of schoolwork?

How did it make you feel?

The North Vietnamese Army was fighting in a civil war.

China's neighbor, North Vietnam, was at war with South Vietnam and the United States. North Vietnam asked China for help preventing malaria in its army. The disease was making lots of soldiers sick or even killing them. China's leader, Mao Zedong, launched Project 523 to find a cure for malaria. In 1969, Tu took charge of the project.

Mao Zedong

Tu visited the rain forests of Hainan Island, which had very high levels of malaria.

Scientists around the world had tested more than 240,000 compounds against malaria, but none worked. Tu and her team studied ancient medical texts to learn how people used to fight malaria. Eventually they learned that a plant named sweet wormwood was used to treat fevers in about 400 CE.

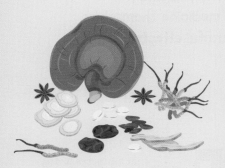

Did You Know?

Vaccines teach our bodies to fight a dead or weakened version of the germ that causes a disease. This triggers the body's natural immune system to make antibodies. The antibodies attach themselves to germs so the immune system can identify them and kill them.

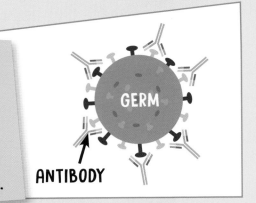

GERM

ANTIBODY

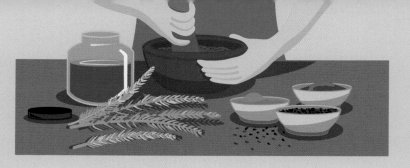

Fevers are a symptom of malaria, so this was a promising clue. In 1971, Tu's team found a compound in sweet wormwood that prevented malaria in animals. The compound was called artemisinin. Before they gave it to patients, Tu and her colleagues took the medicine themselves to check if it had harmful effects.

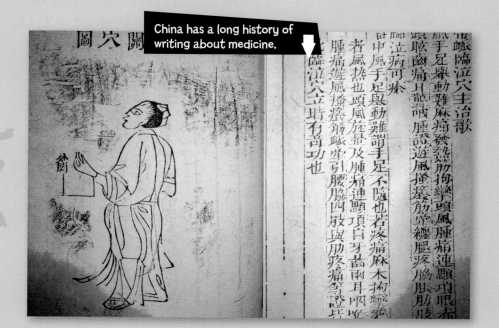

China has a long history of writing about medicine.

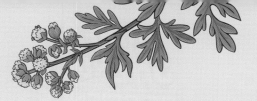

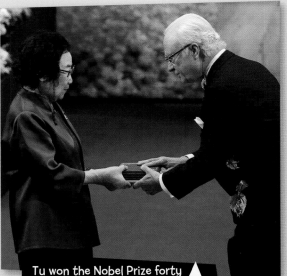

Tu won the Nobel Prize forty years after her discovery.

It was another two decades before Tu's work became known across the world. In the 2000s, the World Health Organization (WHO) finally recommended that artemisinin be used as a treatment for malaria. Tu's discovery has saved many lives from malaria around the world. In 2015, Tu won the Nobel Prize for Medicine. **Her breakthrough is still not well known compared with its huge impact on people's lives.**

What Would You Do?

Tu and her team tested artemisinin on themselves before trying it on others. It was a brave act to take, because no one knew if the medicine would have side effects on humans that were worse than malaria itself.

If you were a scientist, would you be happy to test a new medicine on yourself?

If so, why?   If not, why not?

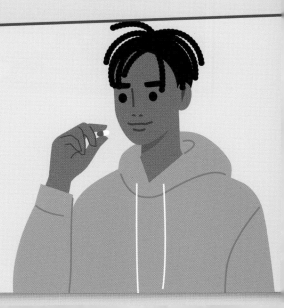

Improving
Health
NURSING

Florence Nightingale

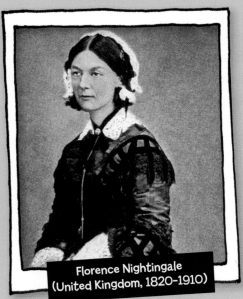

Florence Nightingale
(United Kingdom, 1820-1910)

Florence Nightingale trained as a nurse against the wishes of her wealthy family because she wanted to help others. During the Crimean War (1853-56) against Russia, more soldiers died from disease than in battle. Florence took volunteer nurses to run a British army hospital in Turkey, where wounded soldiers recovered. She realized that hygiene helped stop the spread of infectious diseases. She made sure wards were kept clean and the windows were opened for fresh air. This cut the death rate by two-thirds. She became famous as "the lady with the lamp" for touring the wards at night. Florence went on to set up training programs for nurses and lay the foundations for modern nursing.

Dorothy Hodgkin

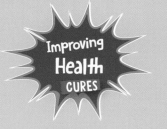

Dorothy Hodgkin did her first chemistry experiments when she was just fourteen. As a scientist, she developed a way to use **X-rays** to photograph the structure of chemicals found in living things, which she used to help improve medicines. She mapped the **molecular** structure of penicillin, an antibiotic medicine that treats infections. It took her thirty-five years to map the structure of **insulin**, which is used to treat diabetes, a disease that affects how the body uses sugar. Dorothy won the Nobel Prize for Chemistry in 1964.

Dorothy Hodgkin
(United Kingdom, 1910–1994)

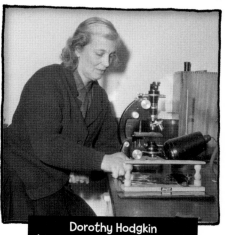

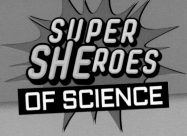

SUPER SHEROES OF SCIENCE

Improving **Health** MEDICINE

Susan La Flesche Picotte

Susan La Flesche Picotte, a member of the Omaha tribe, was the first Indigenous woman in the United States to get a degree in medicine. She became a doctor on the Omaha Reservation in Nebraska. She visited the sick on the reservation and campaigned to raise levels of hygiene and sanitation to avoid disease.

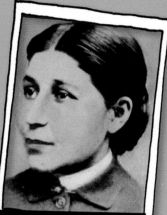

Susan La Flesche Picotte (United States, 1865-1915)

Rosalyn Sussman Yalow

Improving **Health** DISEASES

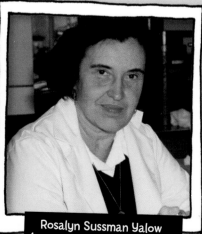

Rosalyn Sussman Yalow (United States, 1921-2011)

Rosalyn Sussman Yalow's parents hoped she would become a teacher, but the New Yorker became a physics professor instead. She helped develop a way of measuring tiny quantities of substances in human blood. This technique made it easier to study the causes of diseases such as diabetes. Rosalyn won the Nobel Prize for Medicine in 1977.

Helen Rodríguez Trías

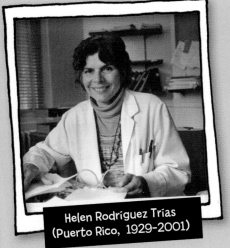

Helen Rodríguez Trías
(Puerto Rico, 1929-2001)

Growing up in Puerto Rico and New York City, Helen Rodríguez Trías became a pediatrician at a time when **discrimination** prevented many Puerto Ricans from studying medicine. She campaigned to improve the medical care available to the poor, particularly children and immigrants. She also worked to improve conditions for people with HIV/AIDS disease.

Elizabeth Blackburn

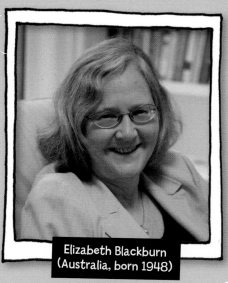

Elizabeth Blackburn
(Australia, born 1948)

Growing up in Australia, Elizabeth Blackburn was fascinated by animals, and went on to study **biochemistry**. She investigated **chromosomes**, opening the way for improved treatments for cancer and a better understanding of why humans age. Elizabeth and her student Carol Greider won the Nobel Prize for Medicine in 2009.

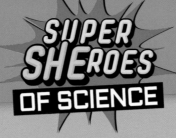

Patricia Bath

When Patricia Bath was young, her mother bought her a chemistry set to encourage her interest in science. Patricia earned a medical degree before studying ophthalmology, or eye care. She looked after her local community in Harlem, New York, where Black people suffered a high level of eye problems. Patricia moved to the University of California at Los Angeles, and introduced new ways to train eye surgeons. She also invented an improved laser to operate on cataracts, a condition that causes blindness around the world. Patricia also helped found the American Institute for the Prevention of Blindness, an organization that promotes visual health.

Improving Health VISION

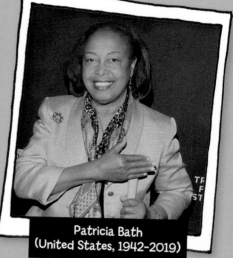

Patricia Bath
(United States, 1942–2019)

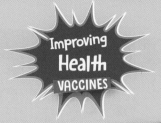

Sarah Gilbert

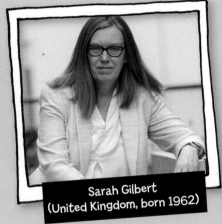

Sarah Gilbert
(United Kingdom, born 1962)

Sarah Gilbert is a vaccinologist, a scientist who works to develop vaccines. During her career, she has developed vaccines for diseases such as malaria, flu, Ebola, and MERS. She has traveled the world to visit disease hot spots. When the COVID-19 **pandemic** began in 2020, Sarah's team developed a vaccine and began to test it. It became one of the first vaccines against COVID-19, produced by the University of Oxford with the company AstraZeneca.

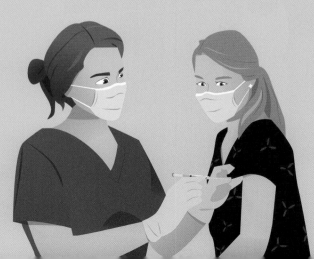

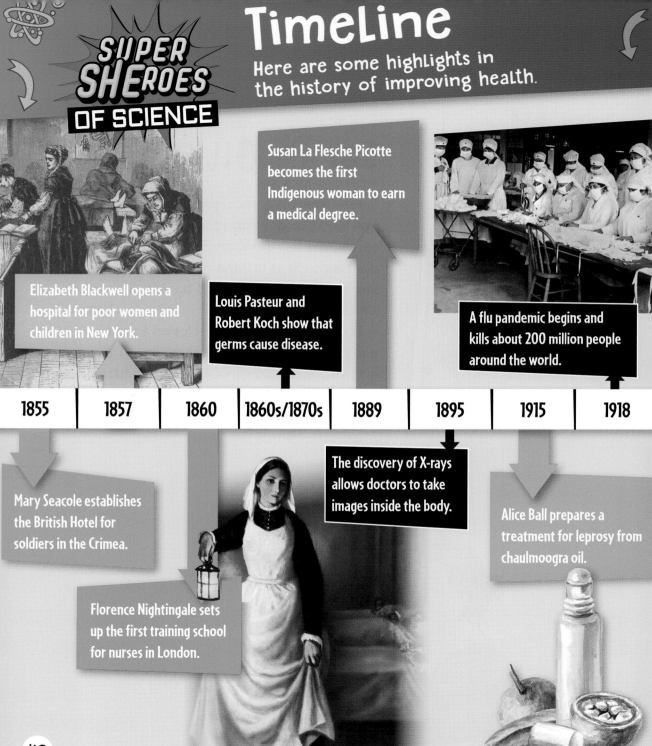

TimeLine

Here are some highlights in the history of improving health.

SUPER SHEROES OF SCIENCE

Susan La Flesche Picotte becomes the first Indigenous woman to earn a medical degree.

Elizabeth Blackwell opens a hospital for poor women and children in New York.

Louis Pasteur and Robert Koch show that germs cause disease.

A flu pandemic begins and kills about 200 million people around the world.

1855	1857	1860	1860s/1870s	1889	1895	1915	1918

Mary Seacole establishes the British Hotel for soldiers in the Crimea.

The discovery of X-rays allows doctors to take images inside the body.

Alice Ball prepares a treatment for leprosy from chaulmoogra oil.

Florence Nightingale sets up the first training school for nurses in London.

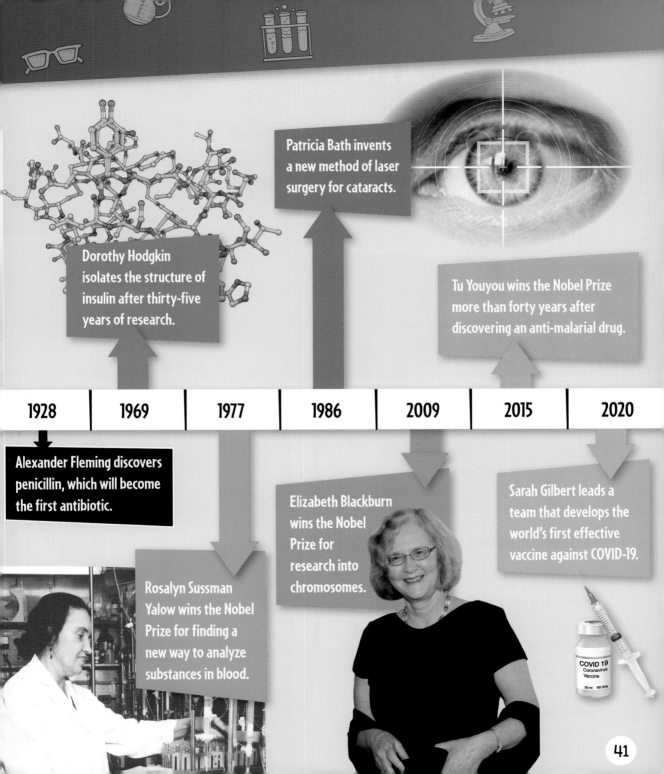

Patricia Bath invents a new method of laser surgery for cataracts.

Dorothy Hodgkin isolates the structure of insulin after thirty-five years of research.

Tu Youyou wins the Nobel Prize more than forty years after discovering an anti-malarial drug.

1928   **1969**   **1977**   **1986**   **2009**   **2015**   **2020**

Alexander Fleming discovers penicillin, which will become the first antibiotic.

Elizabeth Blackburn wins the Nobel Prize for research into chromosomes.

Sarah Gilbert leads a team that develops the world's first effective vaccine against COVID-19.

Rosalyn Sussman Yalow wins the Nobel Prize for finding a new way to analyze substances in blood.

COVID 19
Coronavirus
Vaccine
20 ml   RX Only

1. Alice Ball
Honolulu, Hawaii
Alice spent most of her career at the University of Hawaii in Honolulu.

2. Patricia Bath
Los Angeles
Patricia invented an improved laser to operate on cataracts while working at UCLA.

3. Elizabeth Blackburn
Melbourne, Australia
Elizabeth got her degree in science at the University of Melbourne.

4. Elizabeth Blackwell
New York
Elizabeth set up a hospital to care for poor women and children in Lower Manhattan.

5. Sarah Gilbert
Oxford, United Kingdom
Sarah led the team developing COVID vaccines at the University of Oxford.

6. Dorothy Hodgkin
Oxford, United Kingdom
Dorothy spent most of her life working in Oxford, where she ran her own laboratory.

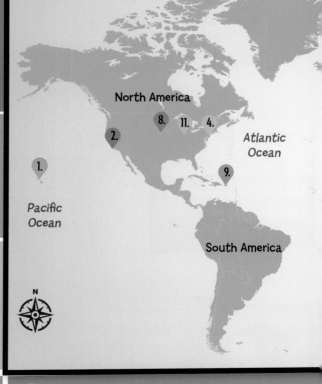

7. Florence Nightingale
Istanbul, Turkey
Florence's hospital was at Scutari, a neighborhood of the Turkish capital, Istanbul.

8. Susan La Flesche Picotte
Omaha Reservation, Nebraska
Susan traveled widely across the Omaha Reservation to visit the sick.

10. Mary Seacole
Crimean Peninsula, Russia
Mary's British Hotel was only a few miles from the front lines in the Crimean War.

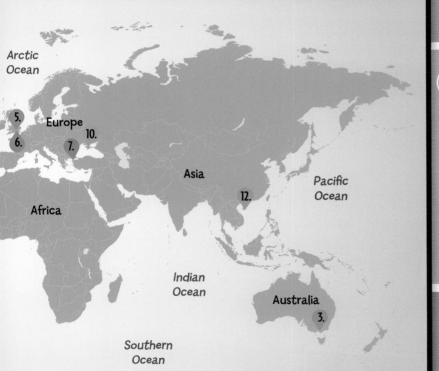

Arctic Ocean

Europe

5.

6.

10.

7.

Asia

12.

Pacific Ocean

Africa

Indian Ocean

Australia

3.

Southern Ocean

11. Rosalyn Sussman Yalow
Champaign, Illinois
When Rosalyn became an assistant professor at the University of Illinois in 1941, she was the only woman among a faculty of 400.

12. Tu Youyou
Hainan Province, China
Tu traveled to China's tropical Hainan Island to study the conditions that helped malaria spread.

9. Helen Rodríguez Trías
San Juan, Puerto Rico
Helen noticed in her early jobs that women from her native Puerto Rico were not well supported by the health system.

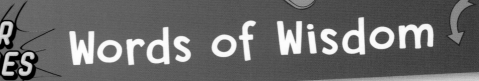

Words of Wisdom

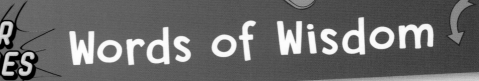

SUPER SHEroes OF SCIENCE

Read the inspirational words of these
Super SHEroes of Science and remember:
You can become a Super SHEro, too!

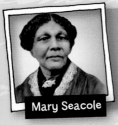

Mary Seacole

" I had from early youth a yearning for medical knowledge
and practice which never deserted me . . . And I was very
young when I began to make use of the little knowledge I had
acquired from watching my mother. "

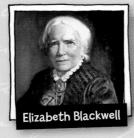

Elizabeth Blackwell

" It is not easy to be a pioneer but oh, it is
fascinating! I would not trade one moment, even
the worst moment, for all the riches in the world. "

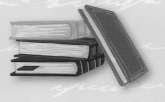

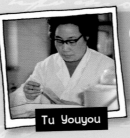

Tu Youyou

" Every scientist dreams
of doing something that can
help the world. "

44

> 66 Believe in the power of truth. Do not allow your mind to be imprisoned by majority thinking. Remember that the limits of science are not the limits of imagination. 99

Patricia Bath

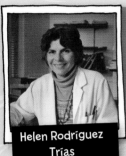

Helen Rodríguez Trías

> 66 We cannot achieve a healthier us without achieving a healthier, more equitable [fairer] health care system, and ultimately, a more equitable [fairer] society. 99

> 66 [Women] must believe in ourselves or no one else will believe in us; we must match our aspirations with the guts and determination to succeed. 99

Rosalyn Sussman Yalow

> 66 Why are we even discussing women scientists? I'm not a woman scientist, I'm a scientist and more than half my colleagues are women and we do the job. 99

Sarah Gilbert

45

Glossary

antibodies (**an**-ti-*bah*-deez) proteins made in the blood to stop infections in the body

biochemistry (*bye*-oh-**kem**-i-stree) the study of the chemicals in living things

chemistry (**kem**-i-stree) the study of the makeup of substances and how they react with one another

chromosomes (**kroh**-muh-*sohmz*) structures inside cell nuclei that carry genes

compound (**kahm**-*pound*) a substance made from two or more chemical elements

discrimination (dis-*krim*-i-**nay**-shuhn) unfair treatment of others based on differences in things such as gender or race

epidemics (ep-i-**dem**-iks) diseases that are present in a large number of people at the same time

herbal (urb-uhl) related to plants

hygiene (**hye**-jeen) keeping yourself and your surroundings clean in order to stay healthy

immune system (i-**myoon sis**-tuhm) the system that protects the body against disease and infection

infectious (in-**fek**-shuhs) spreads easily from one person to another

insulin (**in**-suh-lin) a substance that controls the level of sugar in the blood

isolate (**eye**-suh-*late*) to identify the part of a substance that has a particular effect

laser (**lay**-zur) a device that produces a very thin, powerful beam of light

microbes (**mye**-krobz) tiny living things that cause disease

molecular (muh-**lek**-yuh-lur) related to molecules, the smallest units of a chemical compound

pandemic (pan-**dem**-ik) an outbreak of disease that affects a very large area or the whole world

peninsula (puh-**nin**-suh-luh) a piece of land that is almost completely surrounded by water

symptoms (**simp**-tuhmz) signs of illness

vaccines (vak-**seenz**) substances that cause the body to produce antibodies to protect it from disease

X-rays (eks-**rayz**) invisible beams of light used to take pictures of the insides of objects

Index

Further Reading

Ignotofsky, Rachel. *Women in Science: 50 Fearless Pioneers Who Changed the World.* New York: Crown Books for Young Readers, 2021.

Orr, Tamra B. *Antibiotics* (True Books). New York: Scholastic, 2016.

Shea, John. *Bitten! Mosquitoes Infect New York.* (XBooks: Medical). New York: Scholastic, 2020.

Tilden, Thomasine E. Lewis. *Dangerous Worms: Parasites Plague a Village* (XBooks: Medical). New York: Scholastic, 2020.

About the Author

Anita Dalal grew up in an Anglo-Indian family in northern England. She studied for her PhD in London and traveled widely around the world, including many visits with her family in India, before settling in London with her own family. She has written many books for children, often about history and geography. She loved learning new facts about some of her scientific heroines for this book—and discovering other Super SHEroes of Science for the first time! When she's not in the library or at her desk working, she spends her time gardening, walking Monty the golden Labrador, and watching her son play sports. She loves swimming outdoors—even when it's freezing!

About the Consultant

Isabel Thomas is a science communicator and American Association for the Advancement of Science award-winning author. She has degrees in Human Sciences from the University of Oxford and in Education Research from the University of Cambridge, where her academic research focused on addressing inequalities in aspiration and access to science education and careers.